VETERINARY MEDICAL CASE LOG

THIS BOOK BELONGS TO:

HOW TO USE THIS BOOK

This book was created for veterinarians, vet techs, and students to efficiently document important information about their medical cases. Interns and residents can use this book to track patients treated during their programs.

Use the blank lined pages for additional notes about each patient. Case details may be recorded on both sides of the same page, or side by side allowing all information to be seen when the book is laid flat.

Use the check boxes to ensure that all tasks associated with a case are complete.

Be efficient and organized.

DATE: ID#:

PATIENT NAME:

AGE: GENDER:

SPECIES/BREED:

HISTORY:

DIAGNOSIS/PROBLEM LIST:

TREATMENTS/PROCEDURES:

NOTES:

DIAGNOTICS:

- [ ] Blood Work
- [ ] Radiographs
- [ ] Urinalysis
- [ ]
- [ ]
- [ ]

TO DO:

- [ ] Medical Record Complete
- [ ] Outside Lab Diagnostics
- [ ] Follow up call/appointment
- [ ]
- [ ]
- [ ]

DATE: ID#:

PATIENT NAME:

AGE: GENDER:

SPECIES/BREED:

HISTORY:

DIAGNOSIS/PROBLEM LIST:

TREATMENTS/PROCEDURES:

NOTES:

DIAGNOTICS:

- [ ] Blood Work
- [ ] Radiographs
- [ ] Urinalysis
- [ ]
- [ ]
- [ ]

TO DO:

- [ ] Medical Record Complete
- [ ] Outside Lab Diagnostics
- [ ] Follow up call/appointment
- [ ]
- [ ]
- [ ]

DATE: ID#:

PATIENT NAME:

AGE: GENDER:

SPECIES/BREED:

HISTORY:

DIAGNOSIS/PROBLEM LIST:

TREATMENTS/PROCEDURES:

NOTES:

DIAGNOTICS:

- [ ] Blood Work
- [ ] Radiographs
- [ ] Urinalysis
- [ ]
- [ ]
- [ ]

TO DO:

- [ ] Medical Record Complete
- [ ] Outside Lab Diagnostics
- [ ] Follow up call/appointment
- [ ]
- [ ]
- [ ]

DATE: ID#:

PATIENT NAME:

AGE: GENDER:

SPECIES/BREED:

HISTORY:

DIAGNOSIS/PROBLEM LIST:

TREATMENTS/PROCEDURES:

NOTES:

DIAGNOTICS:

- [ ] Blood Work
- [ ] Radiographs
- [ ] Urinalysis
- [ ]
- [ ]
- [ ]

TO DO:

- [ ] Medical Record Complete
- [ ] Outside Lab Diagnostics
- [ ] Follow up call/appointment
- [ ]
- [ ]
- [ ]

DATE: ID#:

PATIENT NAME:

AGE: GENDER:

SPECIES/BREED:

HISTORY:

DIAGNOSIS/PROBLEM LIST:

TREATMENTS/PROCEDURES:

NOTES:

DIAGNOTICS:

- [ ] Blood Work
- [ ] Radiographs
- [ ] Urinalysis
- [ ]
- [ ]
- [ ]

TO DO:

- [ ] Medical Record Complete
- [ ] Outside Lab Diagnostics
- [ ] Follow up call/appointment
- [ ]
- [ ]
- [ ]

DATE: ID#:

PATIENT NAME:

AGE: GENDER:

SPECIES/BREED:

HISTORY:

DIAGNOSIS/PROBLEM LIST:

TREATMENTS/PROCEDURES:

NOTES:

DIAGNOTICS:

- [ ] Blood Work
- [ ] Radiographs
- [ ] Urinalysis
- [ ]
- [ ]
- [ ]

TO DO:

- [ ] Medical Record Complete
- [ ] Outside Lab Diagnostics
- [ ] Follow up call/appointment
- [ ]
- [ ]
- [ ]

DATE: ID#:

PATIENT NAME:

AGE: GENDER:

SPECIES/BREED:

HISTORY:

DIAGNOSIS/PROBLEM LIST:

TREATMENTS/PROCEDURES:

NOTES:

DIAGNOTICS:

- [ ] Blood Work
- [ ] Radiographs
- [ ] Urinalysis
- [ ]
- [ ]
- [ ]

TO DO:

- [ ] Medical Record Complete
- [ ] Outside Lab Diagnostics
- [ ] Follow up call/appointment
- [ ]
- [ ]
- [ ]

DATE: ID#:

PATIENT NAME:

AGE: GENDER:

SPECIES/BREED:

HISTORY:

DIAGNOSIS/PROBLEM LIST:

TREATMENTS/PROCEDURES:

NOTES:

DIAGNOTICS:

- [ ] Blood Work
- [ ] Radiographs
- [ ] Urinalysis
- [ ]
- [ ]
- [ ]

TO DO:

- [ ] Medical Record Complete
- [ ] Outside Lab Diagnostics
- [ ] Follow up call/appointment
- [ ]
- [ ]
- [ ]

DATE: ID#:

PATIENT NAME:

AGE: GENDER:

SPECIES/BREED:

HISTORY:

DIAGNOSIS/PROBLEM LIST:

TREATMENTS/PROCEDURES:

NOTES:

DIAGNOTICS:

- [ ] Blood Work
- [ ] Radiographs
- [ ] Urinalysis
- [ ]
- [ ]
- [ ]

TO DO:

- [ ] Medical Record Complete
- [ ] Outside Lab Diagnostics
- [ ] Follow up call/appointment
- [ ]
- [ ]
- [ ]

DATE: ID#:

PATIENT NAME:

AGE: GENDER:

SPECIES/BREED:

HISTORY:

DIAGNOSIS/PROBLEM LIST:

TREATMENTS/PROCEDURES:

NOTES:

DIAGNOTICS:

- [ ] Blood Work
- [ ] Radiographs
- [ ] Urinalysis
- [ ]
- [ ]
- [ ]

TO DO:

- [ ] Medical Record Complete
- [ ] Outside Lab Diagnostics
- [ ] Follow up call/appointment
- [ ]
- [ ]
- [ ]

DATE: ID#:

PATIENT NAME:

AGE: GENDER:

SPECIES/BREED:

HISTORY:

DIAGNOSIS/PROBLEM LIST:

TREATMENTS/PROCEDURES:

NOTES:

DIAGNOTICS:

- [ ] Blood Work
- [ ] Radiographs
- [ ] Urinalysis
- [ ]
- [ ]
- [ ]

TO DO:

- [ ] Medical Record Complete
- [ ] Outside Lab Diagnostics
- [ ] Follow up call/appointment
- [ ]
- [ ]
- [ ]

DATE: ID#:

PATIENT NAME:

AGE: GENDER:

SPECIES/BREED:

HISTORY:

DIAGNOSIS/PROBLEM LIST:

TREATMENTS/PROCEDURES:

NOTES:

DIAGNOTICS:

- [ ] Blood Work
- [ ] Radiographs
- [ ] Urinalysis
- [ ]
- [ ]
- [ ]

TO DO:

- [ ] Medical Record Complete
- [ ] Outside Lab Diagnostics
- [ ] Follow up call/appointment
- [ ]
- [ ]
- [ ]

DATE: ID#:

PATIENT NAME:

AGE: GENDER:

SPECIES/BREED:

HISTORY:

DIAGNOSIS/PROBLEM LIST:

TREATMENTS/PROCEDURES:

NOTES:

DIAGNOTICS:

- [ ] Blood Work
- [ ] Radiographs
- [ ] Urinalysis
- [ ]
- [ ]
- [ ]

TO DO:

- [ ] Medical Record Complete
- [ ] Outside Lab Diagnostics
- [ ] Follow up call/appointment
- [ ]
- [ ]
- [ ]

DATE: ID#:

PATIENT NAME:

AGE: GENDER:

SPECIES/BREED:

HISTORY:

DIAGNOSIS/PROBLEM LIST:

TREATMENTS/PROCEDURES:

NOTES:

DIAGNOTICS:

- [ ] Blood Work
- [ ] Radiographs
- [ ] Urinalysis
- [ ]
- [ ]
- [ ]

TO DO:

- [ ] Medical Record Complete
- [ ] Outside Lab Diagnostics
- [ ] Follow up call/appointment
- [ ]
- [ ]
- [ ]

DATE: ID#:

PATIENT NAME:

AGE: GENDER:

SPECIES/BREED:

HISTORY:

DIAGNOSIS/PROBLEM LIST:

TREATMENTS/PROCEDURES:

NOTES:

DIAGNOTICS:

- [ ] Blood Work
- [ ] Radiographs
- [ ] Urinalysis
- [ ]
- [ ]
- [ ]

TO DO:

- [ ] Medical Record Complete
- [ ] Outside Lab Diagnostics
- [ ] Follow up call/appointment
- [ ]
- [ ]
- [ ]

DATE: ID#:

PATIENT NAME:

AGE: GENDER:

SPECIES/BREED:

HISTORY:

DIAGNOSIS/PROBLEM LIST:

TREATMENTS/PROCEDURES:

NOTES:

DIAGNOTICS:

- [ ] Blood Work
- [ ] Radiographs
- [ ] Urinalysis
- [ ]
- [ ]
- [ ]

TO DO:

- [ ] Medical Record Complete
- [ ] Outside Lab Diagnostics
- [ ] Follow up call/appointment
- [ ]
- [ ]
- [ ]

DATE: ID#:

PATIENT NAME:

AGE: GENDER:

SPECIES/BREED:

HISTORY:

DIAGNOSIS/PROBLEM LIST:

TREATMENTS/PROCEDURES:

NOTES:

DIAGNOTICS:

- [ ] Blood Work
- [ ] Radiographs
- [ ] Urinalysis
- [ ]
- [ ]
- [ ]

TO DO:

- [ ] Medical Record Complete
- [ ] Outside Lab Diagnostics
- [ ] Follow up call/appointment
- [ ]
- [ ]
- [ ]

DATE: ID#:

PATIENT NAME:

AGE: GENDER:

SPECIES/BREED:

HISTORY:

DIAGNOSIS/PROBLEM LIST:

TREATMENTS/PROCEDURES:

NOTES:

DIAGNOTICS:

- [ ] Blood Work
- [ ] Radiographs
- [ ] Urinalysis
- [ ]
- [ ]
- [ ]

TO DO:

- [ ] Medical Record Complete
- [ ] Outside Lab Diagnostics
- [ ] Follow up call/appointment
- [ ]
- [ ]
- [ ]

DATE: ID#:

PATIENT NAME:

AGE: GENDER:

SPECIES/BREED:

HISTORY:

DIAGNOSIS/PROBLEM LIST:

TREATMENTS/PROCEDURES:

NOTES:

DIAGNOTICS:

- [ ] Blood Work
- [ ] Radiographs
- [ ] Urinalysis
- [ ]
- [ ]
- [ ]

TO DO:

- [ ] Medical Record Complete
- [ ] Outside Lab Diagnostics
- [ ] Follow up call/appointment
- [ ]
- [ ]
- [ ]

DATE: ID#:

PATIENT NAME:

AGE: GENDER:

SPECIES/BREED:

HISTORY:

DIAGNOSIS/PROBLEM LIST:

TREATMENTS/PROCEDURES:

NOTES:

DIAGNOTICS:

- ☐ Blood Work
- ☐ Radiographs
- ☐ Urinalysis
- ☐
- ☐
- ☐

TO DO:

- ☐ Medical Record Complete
- ☐ Outside Lab Diagnostics
- ☐ Follow up call/appointment
- ☐
- ☐
- ☐

DATE: ID#:

PATIENT NAME:

AGE: GENDER:

SPECIES/BREED:

HISTORY:

DIAGNOSIS/PROBLEM LIST:

TREATMENTS/PROCEDURES:

NOTES:

DIAGNOTICS:

- [ ] Blood Work
- [ ] Radiographs
- [ ] Urinalysis
- [ ]
- [ ]
- [ ]

TO DO:

- [ ] Medical Record Complete
- [ ] Outside Lab Diagnostics
- [ ] Follow up call/appointment
- [ ]
- [ ]
- [ ]

DATE: ID#:

PATIENT NAME:

AGE: GENDER:

SPECIES/BREED:

HISTORY:

DIAGNOSIS/PROBLEM LIST:

TREATMENTS/PROCEDURES:

NOTES:

DIAGNOTICS:

- [ ] Blood Work
- [ ] Radiographs
- [ ] Urinalysis
- [ ]
- [ ]
- [ ]

TO DO:

- [ ] Medical Record Complete
- [ ] Outside Lab Diagnostics
- [ ] Follow up call/appointment
- [ ]
- [ ]
- [ ]

DATE: ID#:

PATIENT NAME:

AGE: GENDER:

SPECIES/BREED:

HISTORY:

DIAGNOSIS/PROBLEM LIST:

TREATMENTS/PROCEDURES:

NOTES:

DIAGNOTICS:

- [ ] Blood Work
- [ ] Radiographs
- [ ] Urinalysis
- [ ]
- [ ]
- [ ]

TO DO:

- [ ] Medical Record Complete
- [ ] Outside Lab Diagnostics
- [ ] Follow up call/appointment
- [ ]
- [ ]
- [ ]

DATE: ID#:

PATIENT NAME:

AGE: GENDER:

SPECIES/BREED:

HISTORY:

DIAGNOSIS/PROBLEM LIST:

TREATMENTS/PROCEDURES:

NOTES:

DIAGNOTICS:

- [ ] Blood Work
- [ ] Radiographs
- [ ] Urinalysis
- [ ]
- [ ]
- [ ]

TO DO:

- [ ] Medical Record Complete
- [ ] Outside Lab Diagnostics
- [ ] Follow up call/appointment
- [ ]
- [ ]
- [ ]

DATE: ID#:

PATIENT NAME:

AGE: GENDER:

SPECIES/BREED:

HISTORY:

DIAGNOSIS/PROBLEM LIST:

TREATMENTS/PROCEDURES:

NOTES:

DIAGNOTICS:

- [ ] Blood Work
- [ ] Radiographs
- [ ] Urinalysis
- [ ]
- [ ]
- [ ]

TO DO:

- [ ] Medical Record Complete
- [ ] Outside Lab Diagnostics
- [ ] Follow up call/appointment
- [ ]
- [ ]
- [ ]

DATE: ID#:

PATIENT NAME:

AGE: GENDER:

SPECIES/BREED:

HISTORY:

DIAGNOSIS/PROBLEM LIST:

TREATMENTS/PROCEDURES:

NOTES:

DIAGNOTICS:

- [ ] Blood Work
- [ ] Radiographs
- [ ] Urinalysis
- [ ]
- [ ]
- [ ]

TO DO:

- [ ] Medical Record Complete
- [ ] Outside Lab Diagnostics
- [ ] Follow up call/appointment
- [ ]
- [ ]
- [ ]

DATE: ID#:

PATIENT NAME:

AGE: GENDER:

SPECIES/BREED:

HISTORY:

DIAGNOSIS/PROBLEM LIST:

TREATMENTS/PROCEDURES:

NOTES:

DIAGNOTICS:

- [ ] Blood Work
- [ ] Radiographs
- [ ] Urinalysis
- [ ]
- [ ]
- [ ]

TO DO:

- [ ] Medical Record Complete
- [ ] Outside Lab Diagnostics
- [ ] Follow up call/appointment
- [ ]
- [ ]
- [ ]

DATE: ID#:

PATIENT NAME:

AGE: GENDER:

SPECIES/BREED:

HISTORY:

DIAGNOSIS/PROBLEM LIST:

TREATMENTS/PROCEDURES:

NOTES:

DIAGNOTICS:

- [ ] Blood Work
- [ ] Radiographs
- [ ] Urinalysis
- [ ]
- [ ]
- [ ]

TO DO:

- [ ] Medical Record Complete
- [ ] Outside Lab Diagnostics
- [ ] Follow up call/appointment
- [ ]
- [ ]
- [ ]

DATE: ID#:

PATIENT NAME:

AGE: GENDER:

SPECIES/BREED:

HISTORY:

DIAGNOSIS/PROBLEM LIST:

TREATMENTS/PROCEDURES:

NOTES:

DIAGNOTICS:

- [ ] Blood Work
- [ ] Radiographs
- [ ] Urinalysis
- [ ]
- [ ]
- [ ]

TO DO:

- [ ] Medical Record Complete
- [ ] Outside Lab Diagnostics
- [ ] Follow up call/appointment
- [ ]
- [ ]
- [ ]

DATE: ID#:

PATIENT NAME:

AGE: GENDER:

SPECIES/BREED:

HISTORY:

DIAGNOSIS/PROBLEM LIST:

TREATMENTS/PROCEDURES:

NOTES:

DIAGNOTICS:

- [ ] Blood Work
- [ ] Radiographs
- [ ] Urinalysis
- [ ]
- [ ]
- [ ]

TO DO:

- [ ] Medical Record Complete
- [ ] Outside Lab Diagnostics
- [ ] Follow up call/appointment
- [ ]
- [ ]
- [ ]

DATE: ID#:

PATIENT NAME:

AGE: GENDER:

SPECIES/BREED:

HISTORY:

DIAGNOSIS/PROBLEM LIST:

TREATMENTS/PROCEDURES:

NOTES:

DIAGNOTICS:

- [ ] Blood Work
- [ ] Radiographs
- [ ] Urinalysis
- [ ]
- [ ]
- [ ]

TO DO:

- [ ] Medical Record Complete
- [ ] Outside Lab Diagnostics
- [ ] Follow up call/appointment
- [ ]
- [ ]
- [ ]

DATE: ID#:

PATIENT NAME:

AGE: GENDER:

SPECIES/BREED:

HISTORY:

DIAGNOSIS/PROBLEM LIST:

TREATMENTS/PROCEDURES:

NOTES:

DIAGNOTICS:

- [ ] Blood Work
- [ ] Radiographs
- [ ] Urinalysis
- [ ]
- [ ]
- [ ]

TO DO:

- [ ] Medical Record Complete
- [ ] Outside Lab Diagnostics
- [ ] Follow up call/appointment
- [ ]
- [ ]
- [ ]

DATE: ID#:

PATIENT NAME:

AGE: GENDER:

SPECIES/BREED:

HISTORY:

DIAGNOSIS/PROBLEM LIST:

TREATMENTS/PROCEDURES:

NOTES:

DIAGNOTICS:

- [ ] Blood Work
- [ ] Radiographs
- [ ] Urinalysis
- [ ]
- [ ]
- [ ]

TO DO:

- [ ] Medical Record Complete
- [ ] Outside Lab Diagnostics
- [ ] Follow up call/appointment
- [ ]
- [ ]
- [ ]

DATE: ID#:

PATIENT NAME:

AGE: GENDER:

SPECIES/BREED:

HISTORY:

DIAGNOSIS/PROBLEM LIST:

TREATMENTS/PROCEDURES:

NOTES:

DIAGNOTICS:

- [ ] Blood Work
- [ ] Radiographs
- [ ] Urinalysis
- [ ]
- [ ]
- [ ]

TO DO:

- [ ] Medical Record Complete
- [ ] Outside Lab Diagnostics
- [ ] Follow up call/appointment
- [ ]
- [ ]
- [ ]

DATE: ID#:

PATIENT NAME:

AGE: GENDER:

SPECIES/BREED:

HISTORY:

DIAGNOSIS/PROBLEM LIST:

TREATMENTS/PROCEDURES:

NOTES:

DIAGNOTICS:

- [ ] Blood Work
- [ ] Radiographs
- [ ] Urinalysis
- [ ]
- [ ]
- [ ]

TO DO:

- [ ] Medical Record Complete
- [ ] Outside Lab Diagnostics
- [ ] Follow up call/appointment
- [ ]
- [ ]
- [ ]

DATE: ID#:

PATIENT NAME:

AGE: GENDER:

SPECIES/BREED:

HISTORY:

DIAGNOSIS/PROBLEM LIST:

TREATMENTS/PROCEDURES:

NOTES:

DIAGNOTICS:

- [ ] Blood Work
- [ ] Radiographs
- [ ] Urinalysis
- [ ]
- [ ]
- [ ]

TO DO:

- [ ] Medical Record Complete
- [ ] Outside Lab Diagnostics
- [ ] Follow up call/appointment
- [ ]
- [ ]
- [ ]

DATE: ID#:

PATIENT NAME:

AGE: GENDER:

SPECIES/BREED:

HISTORY:

DIAGNOSIS/PROBLEM LIST:

TREATMENTS/PROCEDURES:

NOTES:

DIAGNOTICS:

- ☐ Blood Work
- ☐ Radiographs
- ☐ Urinalysis
- ☐
- ☐
- ☐

TO DO:

- ☐ Medical Record Complete
- ☐ Outside Lab Diagnostics
- ☐ Follow up call/appointment
- ☐
- ☐
- ☐

DATE: ID#:

PATIENT NAME:

AGE: GENDER:

SPECIES/BREED:

HISTORY:

DIAGNOSIS/PROBLEM LIST:

TREATMENTS/PROCEDURES:

NOTES:

DIAGNOTICS:

- [ ] Blood Work
- [ ] Radiographs
- [ ] Urinalysis
- [ ]
- [ ]
- [ ]

TO DO:

- [ ] Medical Record Complete
- [ ] Outside Lab Diagnostics
- [ ] Follow up call/appointment
- [ ]
- [ ]
- [ ]

DATE: ID#:

PATIENT NAME:

AGE: GENDER:

SPECIES/BREED:

HISTORY:

DIAGNOSIS/PROBLEM LIST:

TREATMENTS/PROCEDURES:

NOTES:

DIAGNOTICS:

- [ ] Blood Work
- [ ] Radiographs
- [ ] Urinalysis
- [ ]
- [ ]
- [ ]

TO DO:

- [ ] Medical Record Complete
- [ ] Outside Lab Diagnostics
- [ ] Follow up call/appointment
- [ ]
- [ ]
- [ ]

DATE: ID#:

PATIENT NAME:

AGE: GENDER:

SPECIES/BREED:

HISTORY:

DIAGNOSIS/PROBLEM LIST:

TREATMENTS/PROCEDURES:

NOTES:

DIAGNOTICS:

- [ ] Blood Work
- [ ] Radiographs
- [ ] Urinalysis
- [ ]
- [ ]
- [ ]

TO DO:

- [ ] Medical Record Complete
- [ ] Outside Lab Diagnostics
- [ ] Follow up call/appointment
- [ ]
- [ ]
- [ ]

DATE: ID#:

PATIENT NAME:

AGE: GENDER:

SPECIES/BREED:

HISTORY:

DIAGNOSIS/PROBLEM LIST:

TREATMENTS/PROCEDURES:

NOTES:

DIAGNOTICS:

- [ ] Blood Work
- [ ] Radiographs
- [ ] Urinalysis
- [ ]
- [ ]
- [ ]

TO DO:

- [ ] Medical Record Complete
- [ ] Outside Lab Diagnostics
- [ ] Follow up call/appointment
- [ ]
- [ ]
- [ ]

DATE: ID#:

PATIENT NAME:

AGE: GENDER:

SPECIES/BREED:

HISTORY:

DIAGNOSIS/PROBLEM LIST:

TREATMENTS/PROCEDURES:

NOTES:

DIAGNOTICS:

- [ ] Blood Work
- [ ] Radiographs
- [ ] Urinalysis
- [ ]
- [ ]
- [ ]

TO DO:

- [ ] Medical Record Complete
- [ ] Outside Lab Diagnostics
- [ ] Follow up call/appointment
- [ ]
- [ ]
- [ ]

DATE: ID#:

PATIENT NAME:

AGE: GENDER:

SPECIES/BREED:

HISTORY:

DIAGNOSIS/PROBLEM LIST:

TREATMENTS/PROCEDURES:

NOTES:

DIAGNOTICS:

- [ ] Blood Work
- [ ] Radiographs
- [ ] Urinalysis
- [ ]
- [ ]
- [ ]

TO DO:

- [ ] Medical Record Complete
- [ ] Outside Lab Diagnostics
- [ ] Follow up call/appointment
- [ ]
- [ ]
- [ ]

DATE: ID#:

PATIENT NAME:

AGE: GENDER:

SPECIES/BREED:

HISTORY:

DIAGNOSIS/PROBLEM LIST:

TREATMENTS/PROCEDURES:

NOTES:

DIAGNOTICS:

- [ ] Blood Work
- [ ] Radiographs
- [ ] Urinalysis
- [ ]
- [ ]
- [ ]

TO DO:

- [ ] Medical Record Complete
- [ ] Outside Lab Diagnostics
- [ ] Follow up call/appointment
- [ ]
- [ ]
- [ ]

DATE: ID#:

PATIENT NAME:

AGE: GENDER:

SPECIES/BREED:

HISTORY:

DIAGNOSIS/PROBLEM LIST:

TREATMENTS/PROCEDURES:

NOTES:

DIAGNOTICS:

- [ ] Blood Work
- [ ] Radiographs
- [ ] Urinalysis
- [ ]
- [ ]
- [ ]

TO DO:

- [ ] Medical Record Complete
- [ ] Outside Lab Diagnostics
- [ ] Follow up call/appointment
- [ ]
- [ ]
- [ ]

DATE: ID#:

PATIENT NAME:

AGE: GENDER:

SPECIES/BREED:

HISTORY:

DIAGNOSIS/PROBLEM LIST:

TREATMENTS/PROCEDURES:

NOTES:

DIAGNOTICS:

- [ ] Blood Work
- [ ] Radiographs
- [ ] Urinalysis
- [ ]
- [ ]
- [ ]

TO DO:

- [ ] Medical Record Complete
- [ ] Outside Lab Diagnostics
- [ ] Follow up call/appointment
- [ ]
- [ ]
- [ ]

DATE: ID#:

PATIENT NAME:

AGE: GENDER:

SPECIES/BREED:

HISTORY:

DIAGNOSIS/PROBLEM LIST:

TREATMENTS/PROCEDURES:

NOTES:

DIAGNOTICS:

- [ ] Blood Work
- [ ] Radiographs
- [ ] Urinalysis
- [ ]
- [ ]
- [ ]

TO DO:

- [ ] Medical Record Complete
- [ ] Outside Lab Diagnostics
- [ ] Follow up call/appointment
- [ ]
- [ ]
- [ ]

DATE: ID#:

PATIENT NAME:

AGE: GENDER:

SPECIES/BREED:

HISTORY:

DIAGNOSIS/PROBLEM LIST:

TREATMENTS/PROCEDURES:

NOTES:

DIAGNOTICS:

- [ ] Blood Work
- [ ] Radiographs
- [ ] Urinalysis
- [ ]
- [ ]
- [ ]

TO DO:

- [ ] Medical Record Complete
- [ ] Outside Lab Diagnostics
- [ ] Follow up call/appointment
- [ ]
- [ ]
- [ ]

DATE: ID#:

PATIENT NAME:

AGE: GENDER:

SPECIES/BREED:

HISTORY:

DIAGNOSIS/PROBLEM LIST:

TREATMENTS/PROCEDURES:

NOTES:

DIAGNOTICS:

- [ ] Blood Work
- [ ] Radiographs
- [ ] Urinalysis
- [ ]
- [ ]
- [ ]

TO DO:

- [ ] Medical Record Complete
- [ ] Outside Lab Diagnostics
- [ ] Follow up call/appointment
- [ ]
- [ ]
- [ ]

DATE: ID#:

PATIENT NAME:

AGE: GENDER:

SPECIES/BREED:

HISTORY:

DIAGNOSIS/PROBLEM LIST:

TREATMENTS/PROCEDURES:

NOTES:

DIAGNOTICS:

- [ ] Blood Work
- [ ] Radiographs
- [ ] Urinalysis
- [ ]
- [ ]
- [ ]

TO DO:

- [ ] Medical Record Complete
- [ ] Outside Lab Diagnostics
- [ ] Follow up call/appointment
- [ ]
- [ ]
- [ ]

DATE: ID#:

PATIENT NAME:

AGE: GENDER:

SPECIES/BREED:

HISTORY:

DIAGNOSIS/PROBLEM LIST:

TREATMENTS/PROCEDURES:

NOTES:

DIAGNOTICS:

- [ ] Blood Work
- [ ] Radiographs
- [ ] Urinalysis
- [ ]
- [ ]
- [ ]

TO DO:

- [ ] Medical Record Complete
- [ ] Outside Lab Diagnostics
- [ ] Follow up call/appointment
- [ ]
- [ ]
- [ ]

DATE: ID#:

PATIENT NAME:

AGE: GENDER:

SPECIES/BREED:

HISTORY:

DIAGNOSIS/PROBLEM LIST:

TREATMENTS/PROCEDURES:

NOTES:

DIAGNOTICS:

- [ ] Blood Work
- [ ] Radiographs
- [ ] Urinalysis
- [ ]
- [ ]
- [ ]

TO DO:

- [ ] Medical Record Complete
- [ ] Outside Lab Diagnostics
- [ ] Follow up call/appointment
- [ ]
- [ ]
- [ ]

DATE: ID#:

PATIENT NAME:

AGE: GENDER:

SPECIES/BREED:

HISTORY:

DIAGNOSIS/PROBLEM LIST:

TREATMENTS/PROCEDURES:

NOTES:

DIAGNOTICS:

- [ ] Blood Work
- [ ] Radiographs
- [ ] Urinalysis
- [ ]
- [ ]
- [ ]

TO DO:

- [ ] Medical Record Complete
- [ ] Outside Lab Diagnostics
- [ ] Follow up call/appointment
- [ ]
- [ ]
- [ ]

DATE: ID#:

PATIENT NAME:

AGE: GENDER:

SPECIES/BREED:

HISTORY:

DIAGNOSIS/PROBLEM LIST:

TREATMENTS/PROCEDURES:

NOTES:

DIAGNOTICS:

- [ ] Blood Work
- [ ] Radiographs
- [ ] Urinalysis
- [ ]
- [ ]
- [ ]

TO DO:

- [ ] Medical Record Complete
- [ ] Outside Lab Diagnostics
- [ ] Follow up call/appointment
- [ ]
- [ ]
- [ ]

DATE: ID#:

PATIENT NAME:

AGE: GENDER:

SPECIES/BREED:

HISTORY:

DIAGNOSIS/PROBLEM LIST:

TREATMENTS/PROCEDURES:

NOTES:

DIAGNOTICS:

- [ ] Blood Work
- [ ] Radiographs
- [ ] Urinalysis
- [ ]
- [ ]
- [ ]

TO DO:

- [ ] Medical Record Complete
- [ ] Outside Lab Diagnostics
- [ ] Follow up call/appointment
- [ ]
- [ ]
- [ ]

DATE: ID#:

PATIENT NAME:

AGE: GENDER:

SPECIES/BREED:

HISTORY:

DIAGNOSIS/PROBLEM LIST:

TREATMENTS/PROCEDURES:

NOTES:

DIAGNOTICS:

- [ ] Blood Work
- [ ] Radiographs
- [ ] Urinalysis
- [ ]
- [ ]
- [ ]

TO DO:

- [ ] Medical Record Complete
- [ ] Outside Lab Diagnostics
- [ ] Follow up call/appointment
- [ ]
- [ ]
- [ ]

DATE: ID#:

PATIENT NAME:

AGE: GENDER:

SPECIES/BREED:

HISTORY:

DIAGNOSIS/PROBLEM LIST:

TREATMENTS/PROCEDURES:

NOTES:

DIAGNOTICS:

- [ ] Blood Work
- [ ] Radiographs
- [ ] Urinalysis
- [ ]
- [ ]
- [ ]

TO DO:

- [ ] Medical Record Complete
- [ ] Outside Lab Diagnostics
- [ ] Follow up call/appointment
- [ ]
- [ ]
- [ ]

DATE: ID#:

PATIENT NAME:

AGE: GENDER:

SPECIES/BREED:

HISTORY:

DIAGNOSIS/PROBLEM LIST:

TREATMENTS/PROCEDURES:

NOTES:

DIAGNOTICS:

- ☐ Blood Work
- ☐ Radiographs
- ☐ Urinalysis
- ☐
- ☐
- ☐

TO DO:

- ☐ Medical Record Complete
- ☐ Outside Lab Diagnostics
- ☐ Follow up call/appointment
- ☐
- ☐
- ☐

DATE: ID#:

PATIENT NAME:

AGE: GENDER:

SPECIES/BREED:

HISTORY:

DIAGNOSIS/PROBLEM LIST:

TREATMENTS/PROCEDURES:

NOTES:

DIAGNOTICS:

- [ ] Blood Work
- [ ] Radiographs
- [ ] Urinalysis
- [ ]
- [ ]
- [ ]

TO DO:

- [ ] Medical Record Complete
- [ ] Outside Lab Diagnostics
- [ ] Follow up call/appointment
- [ ]
- [ ]
- [ ]

DATE: ID#:

PATIENT NAME:

AGE: GENDER:

SPECIES/BREED:

HISTORY:

DIAGNOSIS/PROBLEM LIST:

TREATMENTS/PROCEDURES:

NOTES:

DIAGNOTICS:

- [ ] Blood Work
- [ ] Radiographs
- [ ] Urinalysis
- [ ]
- [ ]
- [ ]

TO DO:

- [ ] Medical Record Complete
- [ ] Outside Lab Diagnostics
- [ ] Follow up call/appointment
- [ ]
- [ ]
- [ ]

DATE: ID#:

PATIENT NAME:

AGE: GENDER:

SPECIES/BREED:

HISTORY:

DIAGNOSIS/PROBLEM LIST:

TREATMENTS/PROCEDURES:

NOTES:

DIAGNOTICS:

- [ ] Blood Work
- [ ] Radiographs
- [ ] Urinalysis
- [ ]
- [ ]
- [ ]

TO DO:

- [ ] Medical Record Complete
- [ ] Outside Lab Diagnostics
- [ ] Follow up call/appointment
- [ ]
- [ ]
- [ ]

DATE: ID#:

PATIENT NAME:

AGE: GENDER:

SPECIES/BREED:

HISTORY:

DIAGNOSIS/PROBLEM LIST:

TREATMENTS/PROCEDURES:

NOTES:

DIAGNOTICS:

- [ ] Blood Work
- [ ] Radiographs
- [ ] Urinalysis
- [ ]
- [ ]
- [ ]

TO DO:

- [ ] Medical Record Complete
- [ ] Outside Lab Diagnostics
- [ ] Follow up call/appointment
- [ ]
- [ ]
- [ ]

DATE: ID#:

PATIENT NAME:

AGE: GENDER:

SPECIES/BREED:

HISTORY:

DIAGNOSIS/PROBLEM LIST:

TREATMENTS/PROCEDURES:

NOTES:

DIAGNOTICS:

- [ ] Blood Work
- [ ] Radiographs
- [ ] Urinalysis
- [ ]
- [ ]
- [ ]

TO DO:

- [ ] Medical Record Complete
- [ ] Outside Lab Diagnostics
- [ ] Follow up call/appointment
- [ ]
- [ ]
- [ ]

DATE: ID#:

PATIENT NAME:

AGE: GENDER:

SPECIES/BREED:

HISTORY:

DIAGNOSIS/PROBLEM LIST:

TREATMENTS/PROCEDURES:

NOTES:

DIAGNOTICS:

- [ ] Blood Work
- [ ] Radiographs
- [ ] Urinalysis
- [ ]
- [ ]
- [ ]

TO DO:

- [ ] Medical Record Complete
- [ ] Outside Lab Diagnostics
- [ ] Follow up call/appointment
- [ ]
- [ ]
- [ ]

DATE: ID#:

PATIENT NAME:

AGE: GENDER:

SPECIES/BREED:

HISTORY:

DIAGNOSIS/PROBLEM LIST:

TREATMENTS/PROCEDURES:

NOTES:

DIAGNOTICS:

- [ ] Blood Work
- [ ] Radiographs
- [ ] Urinalysis
- [ ]
- [ ]
- [ ]

TO DO:

- [ ] Medical Record Complete
- [ ] Outside Lab Diagnostics
- [ ] Follow up call/appointment
- [ ]
- [ ]
- [ ]

DATE: ID#:

PATIENT NAME:

AGE: GENDER:

SPECIES/BREED:

HISTORY:

DIAGNOSIS/PROBLEM LIST:

TREATMENTS/PROCEDURES:

NOTES:

DIAGNOTICS:

- [ ] Blood Work
- [ ] Radiographs
- [ ] Urinalysis
- [ ]
- [ ]
- [ ]

TO DO:

- [ ] Medical Record Complete
- [ ] Outside Lab Diagnostics
- [ ] Follow up call/appointment
- [ ]
- [ ]
- [ ]

DATE: ID#:

PATIENT NAME:

AGE: GENDER:

SPECIES/BREED:

HISTORY:

DIAGNOSIS/PROBLEM LIST:

TREATMENTS/PROCEDURES:

NOTES:

DIAGNOTICS:

- [ ] Blood Work
- [ ] Radiographs
- [ ] Urinalysis
- [ ]
- [ ]
- [ ]

TO DO:

- [ ] Medical Record Complete
- [ ] Outside Lab Diagnostics
- [ ] Follow up call/appointment
- [ ]
- [ ]
- [ ]

DATE: ID#:

PATIENT NAME:

AGE: GENDER:

SPECIES/BREED:

HISTORY:

DIAGNOSIS/PROBLEM LIST:

TREATMENTS/PROCEDURES:

NOTES:

DIAGNOTICS:

- ☐ Blood Work
- ☐ Radiographs
- ☐ Urinalysis
- ☐
- ☐
- ☐

TO DO:

- ☐ Medical Record Complete
- ☐ Outside Lab Diagnostics
- ☐ Follow up call/appointment
- ☐
- ☐
- ☐

DATE: ID#:

PATIENT NAME:

AGE: GENDER:

SPECIES/BREED:

HISTORY:

DIAGNOSIS/PROBLEM LIST:

TREATMENTS/PROCEDURES:

NOTES:

DIAGNOTICS:

- [ ] Blood Work
- [ ] Radiographs
- [ ] Urinalysis
- [ ]
- [ ]
- [ ]

TO DO:

- [ ] Medical Record Complete
- [ ] Outside Lab Diagnostics
- [ ] Follow up call/appointment
- [ ]
- [ ]
- [ ]

DATE: ID#:

PATIENT NAME:

AGE: GENDER:

SPECIES/BREED:

HISTORY:

DIAGNOSIS/PROBLEM LIST:

TREATMENTS/PROCEDURES:

NOTES:

DIAGNOTICS:

- [ ] Blood Work
- [ ] Radiographs
- [ ] Urinalysis
- [ ]
- [ ]
- [ ]

TO DO:

- [ ] Medical Record Complete
- [ ] Outside Lab Diagnostics
- [ ] Follow up call/appointment
- [ ]
- [ ]
- [ ]

DATE: ID#:

PATIENT NAME:

AGE: GENDER:

SPECIES/BREED:

HISTORY:

DIAGNOSIS/PROBLEM LIST:

TREATMENTS/PROCEDURES:

NOTES:

DIAGNOTICS:

- [ ] Blood Work
- [ ] Radiographs
- [ ] Urinalysis
- [ ]
- [ ]
- [ ]

TO DO:

- [ ] Medical Record Complete
- [ ] Outside Lab Diagnostics
- [ ] Follow up call/appointment
- [ ]
- [ ]
- [ ]

DATE: ID#:

PATIENT NAME:

AGE: GENDER:

SPECIES/BREED:

HISTORY:

DIAGNOSIS/PROBLEM LIST:

TREATMENTS/PROCEDURES:

NOTES:

DIAGNOTICS:

- [ ] Blood Work
- [ ] Radiographs
- [ ] Urinalysis
- [ ]
- [ ]
- [ ]

TO DO:

- [ ] Medical Record Complete
- [ ] Outside Lab Diagnostics
- [ ] Follow up call/appointment
- [ ]
- [ ]
- [ ]

DATE: ID#:

PATIENT NAME:

AGE: GENDER:

SPECIES/BREED:

HISTORY:

DIAGNOSIS/PROBLEM LIST:

TREATMENTS/PROCEDURES:

NOTES:

DIAGNOTICS:

- [ ] Blood Work
- [ ] Radiographs
- [ ] Urinalysis
- [ ]
- [ ]
- [ ]

TO DO:

- [ ] Medical Record Complete
- [ ] Outside Lab Diagnostics
- [ ] Follow up call/appointment
- [ ]
- [ ]
- [ ]

DATE: ID#:

PATIENT NAME:

AGE: GENDER:

SPECIES/BREED:

HISTORY:

DIAGNOSIS/PROBLEM LIST:

TREATMENTS/PROCEDURES:

NOTES:

DIAGNOTICS:

- [ ] Blood Work
- [ ] Radiographs
- [ ] Urinalysis
- [ ]
- [ ]
- [ ]

TO DO:

- [ ] Medical Record Complete
- [ ] Outside Lab Diagnostics
- [ ] Follow up call/appointment
- [ ]
- [ ]
- [ ]

DATE: ID#:

PATIENT NAME:

AGE: GENDER:

SPECIES/BREED:

HISTORY:

DIAGNOSIS/PROBLEM LIST:

TREATMENTS/PROCEDURES:

NOTES:

DIAGNOTICS:

- [ ] Blood Work
- [ ] Radiographs
- [ ] Urinalysis
- [ ]
- [ ]
- [ ]

TO DO:

- [ ] Medical Record Complete
- [ ] Outside Lab Diagnostics
- [ ] Follow up call/appointment
- [ ]
- [ ]
- [ ]

DATE: ID#:

PATIENT NAME:

AGE: GENDER:

SPECIES/BREED:

HISTORY:

DIAGNOSIS/PROBLEM LIST:

TREATMENTS/PROCEDURES:

NOTES:

DIAGNOTICS:

- [ ] Blood Work
- [ ] Radiographs
- [ ] Urinalysis
- [ ]
- [ ]
- [ ]

TO DO:

- [ ] Medical Record Complete
- [ ] Outside Lab Diagnostics
- [ ] Follow up call/appointment
- [ ]
- [ ]
- [ ]

DATE: ID#:

PATIENT NAME:

AGE: GENDER:

SPECIES/BREED:

HISTORY:

DIAGNOSIS/PROBLEM LIST:

TREATMENTS/PROCEDURES:

NOTES:

DIAGNOTICS:

- [ ] Blood Work
- [ ] Radiographs
- [ ] Urinalysis
- [ ]
- [ ]
- [ ]

TO DO:

- [ ] Medical Record Complete
- [ ] Outside Lab Diagnostics
- [ ] Follow up call/appointment
- [ ]
- [ ]
- [ ]

DATE: ID#:

PATIENT NAME:

AGE: GENDER:

SPECIES/BREED:

HISTORY:

DIAGNOSIS/PROBLEM LIST:

TREATMENTS/PROCEDURES:

NOTES:

DIAGNOTICS:

- [ ] Blood Work
- [ ] Radiographs
- [ ] Urinalysis
- [ ]
- [ ]
- [ ]

TO DO:

- [ ] Medical Record Complete
- [ ] Outside Lab Diagnostics
- [ ] Follow up call/appointment
- [ ]
- [ ]
- [ ]

DATE: ID#:

PATIENT NAME:

AGE: GENDER:

SPECIES/BREED:

HISTORY:

DIAGNOSIS/PROBLEM LIST:

TREATMENTS/PROCEDURES:

NOTES:

DIAGNOTICS:

- [ ] Blood Work
- [ ] Radiographs
- [ ] Urinalysis
- [ ]
- [ ]
- [ ]

TO DO:

- [ ] Medical Record Complete
- [ ] Outside Lab Diagnostics
- [ ] Follow up call/appointment
- [ ]
- [ ]
- [ ]

DATE: ID#:

PATIENT NAME:

AGE: GENDER:

SPECIES/BREED:

HISTORY:

DIAGNOSIS/PROBLEM LIST:

TREATMENTS/PROCEDURES:

NOTES:

DIAGNOTICS:

- [ ] Blood Work
- [ ] Radiographs
- [ ] Urinalysis
- [ ]
- [ ]
- [ ]

TO DO:

- [ ] Medical Record Complete
- [ ] Outside Lab Diagnostics
- [ ] Follow up call/appointment
- [ ]
- [ ]
- [ ]

Made in the USA
Monee, IL
04 November 2026

67375597R00095